HONEY THERAPY

DEDICATION / ACKNOWLEDGEMENT

This book is dedicated to my grandmother who taught me the beauty of honey and to all the beautiful women out there.

SPECIAL THANKS TO:

My beautician and friend, Allison Pete, thanks for all your contribution.

INTRODUCTION:

"Beauty lies in the eye of the beholder" is a popular saying.

There is nothing more beautiful and appealing that a gorgeous woman. She is a perfection that both men and women admire, women world over are willing to do great many things to be perceived as beautiful.

Honey is a sweet food made by bees using nectar from flowers. Honey has had a long history in human consumption, and is used in various foods and beverages as a sweetener and flavoring. Flavors of honey varies based on the nectar source and various types and graved of honey are available. Honey is a mixture of sugars and other compounds. It has been used by human both orally and topically to treat various ailment including gastric disturbances, ulcers, wounds, and burns.

It also contains antioxidants that could potentially help battle the signs of aging in your body. Legend has it that Cleopatra used honey to moisturize her skin and look beautiful. For those looking for an all-natural, organic way to look beautiful without chemicals, honey is your best friend.

In this book, we are analyzing the various benefit of honey and most importantly several do-it-yourself homemade uses of honey for bringing out the beauty in you.

Table of Contents

CHAPTER 1

OVERALL BENEFITS OF HONEY

Honey is a substance produced by bees from the nectar of plants. It is used as a medicine. It has been clinically proven to have actual nutritional benefits. It also contains antioxidants that could potentially help battle the signs of aging in your body. It the oldest natural sweetener with lots of benefits other than just being sweet in taste.

Beyond the delicious taste of honey, it can be beneficial to our health when consumed, such benefits includes;

- Heart health: Flavonoids and antioxidants contents of honey help to reduce the risk of heart disease and some cancers. It also assists in treatment of disorders such as bacterial gastroenteritis and ulcers.
- All honey is antibacterial and anti-fungal because it contains an enzyme produced by bees that make hydrogen peroxide.
- Honey when consumed with dried figs enhances athletic performance because it is excellent in improving recovery as well as maintaining glycogen levels.
- Honey when added to tea or warm lemon water and consumed, is an effective cough suppressant and it also soothes a sore throat. Two teaspoons of honey before bedtime is good

for children suffering from night-time cough and upper respiratory tract infections.

- Honey, when blended together in herbal preparation, enhances the medicinal value and qualities of those medicines. Honey is believed to improve eyesight, enhance weight loss and cure impotence. It is also helps in treating urinary tract disorders, diarrhea, bronchial asthma and nausea.
- Though honey contains natural sugars, it is not the same as white sugar or any artificial sweeteners. The fusion of fructose and glucose in honey helps the body in regulating blood sugar levels.
- Honey when applied externally, has been proven to be effective in healing wounds and burns
- Honey with its anti-microbial properties is excellent for the skin. It softens, and rejuvenates exhausted skin. Honey is used in many homemade face packs as well as in products available in the market.

HONEY AND BEAUTY

For those looking for an all-natural, organic way to look beautiful without chemicals, honey is your best friend. Legend has it that Cleopatra used honey to moisturize her skin and look beautiful. Honey is all-natural humectants. This means that honey attracts and helps retain skin moisture, hydrating your skin without any artificial chemicals or compounds like commercial moisturizers.

Honey is naturally antibacterial, so it's great for acne treatment and prevention. Its antioxidants properties are great for slowing down aging. Honey is clarifying because it opens up pores making them easy to unclog and because It is extremely moisturizing and soothing, it helps to create a glow.

For those suffering from skin blemishes and acne, Honey has powerful, natural anti-bacterial properties which are naturally soothing, making it the perfect all-natural cleanser to moisturize and purify your complexion.

BEAUTY BENEFITS OF HONEY

"Raw honey is incredible for your skin thanks to its antibacterial properties and hefty serving of skin-saving antioxidants, whether you're looking for an inexpensive DIY solution or a powerful skin treatment, raw honey can help you regain your glow."

NUTRITIONAL PROPERTIES OF HONEY

Honey is known as the miracle cure for skin of all types. It has been used since ancient times for the treatment of cuts, burns and to reduce skin swellings. Honey is not only blessed with powerful skin saving antioxidants but also contains amazing anti-inflammatory which help in soothing and healing your inflamed red acne; antiseptic and antibacterial properties which also help in fighting off acne causing germs and bacteria, staving off more acne and pimples.

Some of the potent nutrients in raw honey include;

- ❖ Vitamin B1: Aid in proper skin functioning and healthy skin.
- ❖ Vitamin B2: Protects skin from free radicals that causes damage to the skin.
- ❖ Vitamin B6: Keeps skin moisturized and healthy and promote new skin cell formation.
- ❖ Vitamin B3: Anti-inflammatory which reduces red skin and acne inflammations as well as moisturizes and hydrates dry skin
- ❖ Vitamin C: Healing topical symptoms such as dry skin and rashes.
- ❖ Zinc: Honey contains antioxidants for moisturized and vibrant skin, equally aid in fighting free radicals activities that cause oxidative stress in skin cells, thereby slowing down the aging process of skin.

CHAPTER 2

51 AMAZING BENEFITS AND USES OF HONEY

Looking good is serious business. Every woman wants to get attention with her look first and foremost. Let us examine where we really need to care for, and how honey can be of help. Let us examine the uses of honey for facial, skin, hair, overall health, acne treatment, and weight loss.

One of the oldest natural cosmetics known to man is honey. For centuries, it has been used on its own or added to other ingredients to make creams, cleansers and tonics to keep the skin and hair soft and in beautiful condition.

When warmed and smoothed over the skin, honey attracts dirt away from the pores. This combined with its natural antiseptic properties make it an ideal cleansing agent.

(A) HONEY FACIAL RECIPES

1. **Honey cleansing water**:

   Dissolve two tablespoons of honey into a liter (or two pints) of warm water and splash over the face and neck for up to 10 minutes then rinse with warm water.

2. **Honey cleanser**

   A mixture of honey and oil (try coconut oil or jojoba oil) to form a balmy texture that is slippery enough to slide across your face, with a dash of cinnamon, turmeric or nutmeg for an aromatic treat, massaged over your face with aid in loosening up heavy makeup and moisturizing your skin at the same time. Note that it should not be used in removing delicate eye makeup.

3. *Honey Firming Face Mask Recipes*

To naturally firm and tone your face, Whisk an egg white with a spoonful of organic honey and gently rub onto your face. Leave this mask on for at least 10 minutes, and then gently rinse off with warm water. Your facial skin will feel smooth and clean while minimizing pores and helping erase the signs of aging

4. **HONEY FACIAL MASK RECIPES**: We will be looking at this using different skin types. The steps and ingredients involved are very popular and easy to prepare. Choose the one that suits your skin type and discover the new you shining through.

Honey Dry Skin Recipes:

People with dry skin should use this honey face mask because it contains amazing ingredients that heal and nourish dehydrated skin. It locks moisture into your skin cells, feeding it with the necessary moisture needed for supple, lubricated skin. If you are suffering from dry or aging skin, make this face mask your companion. It is sure to plump up and moisturize your skin cells and leave you looking fresher and younger than ever before.

Tips
- Use a ripe avocado in this mask so it's easier to mash with a fork.
- Avoid the eye and mouth area when applying the mixture as these are more sensitive compared to other parts of your face and the tightening and stretching of the mask may cause wrinkles.
- Before applying the mask, wash your face with warm water and pat dry with a clean towel or steam your face. This is simply to open up your pores so the nutrients of the mask can sink deep into your skin.

Ingredients for different dry skin facial recipes and their importance: want to get rid of your dry flaky skin, ensure you have the following ingredients in your kitchen.

- ❖ **Avocado**: Rich in healthy fat and vitamin E, the nutritious avocado will help feed and lubricate withered skin, giving it a supple look and feel.
- ❖ **Coconut Oil**: An incredible moisturizer and lubricating agent. Coconut oil is blessed with healthy nutrients that nourish dry skin.
- ❖ **Honey** stimulates and smoothes,
- ❖ **Almond oil** penetrate and moisturize
- ❖ **Yogurt** refines and tightens pores.
- ❖ **Egg Yolk**: The egg yolk equally penetrates and moisturizes as well as helps to lighten the skin.
- ❖ **Wheat germ oil:**

5. Dry Skin Recipe 1

Ingredients:
2 tablespoons of avocado flesh

2 tablespoons honey
1 egg yolk

Preparation: Blend all the ingredients in a blender, or mash by hand in a bowl, using your fingers tips, spread the mask over your face and neck, let it sit for at least 30 minutes and wash off with warm water or wash cloth. Not only does this act as anti aging skin care facial mask it also has a lightening effect.

6. ***Dry Skin Recipe 2***: This also aid in skin hydrating, perfect for dry skin.

Ingredients:

1 teaspoon honey
1 teaspoon coconut oil
1/ 4 ripe avocado

Directions:

In a small mixing bowl, mash ¼ an avocado with the back of a fork or blend if it's more convenient for you. Add 1 teaspoon honey and 1 teaspoon coconut oil and mix thoroughly. Using clean fingers, apply a thick coat of this mixture onto your face, leave it for fifteen minutes and gently scrub off the mask using warm water. Afterwards, splash cold water onto your face to close your pores and pat dry with a towel.

7. ***Dry Skin Recipe 3***

Ingredients
1 tablespoon honey
1 egg yolk

1/2 teaspoon almond oil
1 tablespoon yogurt

Instructions: Put all ingredients into a large bowl and stir until it becomes sticky and thick. Apply on your face and let it sit for 5 minutes and wash off with a mild facial soap. This will leave your face well stimulated, lightened, smooth, finely moisturized, and the pore refines and tightened.

8. **Dry Skin Recipe 4:**

Ingredients:
6oz plain yoghurt
¼oz finely-crushed almonds
2teaspoon honey
2teaspoon wheat germ oil

Preparation: Mix all the ingredients into a smooth paste. Apply and massage the mixture into skin. Keep the mask on for 20 minutes.

9. **Dry Skin Recipe 5:**

Ingredients:
1 egg yolk,
2 tablespoons of clear honey
A handful of fine oatmeal to form a thick paste.

Direction: Mix all and massage gently onto the face and neck. Leave for 15-20 minutes then rinse with warm water.

Honey Normal Skin Recipes:

10.   *Normal Skin Recipe 1*

Ingredient
1 Apple, cored & quartered
2 Tablespoons Honey

Preparation: chop the apple into pieces and drop into a food processor, process into a fine paste, add honey and refrigerate for 10 minutes. Using your fingertips, pat the mixture onto your face lightly until the honey feels tacky. Leave it on for 30 minutes and then rinse.

Honey Oily and Acne Prone Skin Recipes:

Ingredients for diverse oily and Acne prone skin recipes and their importance

- ❖ Cocoa:
- ❖ Papaya:.
- ❖ Honey stimulates and smoothes,
- ❖ Cream:
- ❖ Oatmeal Powder: Oats not only nourishes skin of all types but also gently exfoliates skin, removing dead cells from the skin surface, promoting smooth supple skin as well as absorbs excess sebum from within your pores as it is an absorbent
- ❖ Carrot: Carrots are known to be rich in vitamin A and C. They are also rich in potassium. Vitamin A and C are antioxidants. Honey contains sugar, enzymes, minerals, vitamins and amino acids.

11.   *Oily Skin Recipe 1*

Ingredients:

1/3 cup cocoa
3 teaspoons of heavy cream
1/3 cup ripe papaya
¼ cup honey
3 teaspoons of oatmeal powder

Directions: Mix all ingredients very well, apply on your face and let it sit for 10 minutes, and wash off with warm water. This Facial mask helps heal skin blemishes, nourishes, draws out impurities, balances your skin pH, and leave your skin radiant and soft.

12.   *Oily Skin Recipe 2*

Ingredients:
2 to 3 carrots
4 ½ table spoons of honey

Directions: Boil the carrots until tender and then mash them, pour in honey and refrigerate for 10 minutes. Apply gently to the skin and wait for 10 minutes. Rinse off with cool water.

13.   *Oily skin Recipe 3:*

1 tablespoon of lemon juice,
1 teaspoon of honey
2 egg whites
Whisk together and then spread all over the face, leave for 20 minutes, rinse with warm water and pat dry.

Honey Sensitive Skin Recipes:

Ingredients for different recipes for oily and Acne prone skin and their importance

❖ Banana: Bananas contain vitamin A
❖ Egg: eggs contain lecithin, a natural skin emollient
❖ Honey stimulates and smoothes, honey helps to maintain the skin's natural acid mantle.
❖ Milk:
❖ Oatmeal Powder: Oatmeal is high in nourishing vitamins and minerals; it gently cleanses and heals skin.

14.   Sensitive Skin Recipe 1

Ingredients:
1/2 mashed banana
1/4 cup oatmeal,
Milk
1 egg
1/2 tablespoon honey

Instructions: Mix ingredients together, massage onto face in circular motion and leave on for 15 minutes and rinse with tepid water.

HONEY BEAUTY RECIPE FOR ALL SKIN TYPES:

Ingredients for recipes for all skin types and their importance

❖ Lavender essential oil
❖ Honey stimulates and smoothes,

- ❖ Lemon:
- ❖ Olive, Jojoba or Coconut oil
- ❖ Egg yolk

15. *All skin Recipe 1*

Ingredients
1 tablespoon raw honey
3 drops lavender essential oil

Directions: Stir the ingredients together, dampen your face with warm water, smooth on mixture, let it sit for 15 minutes and wash off with warm water.

16. *All skin Recipe 2 (Skin Lightening effect)*

Ingredients:
1 tablespoon honey
1 teaspoon lemon juice

Directions: Mix the two ingredients thoroughly, apply as a mask and leave on for 20 to30 minutes. Wash off with warm water.

17. *All skin Recipe 3*

1 teaspoon honey (preferably raw honey)
1 teaspoon oil (Olive, Jojoba or Coconut)
Yoke of an egg

Blend all together and apply to face. Leave on for 15-20 minutes and wash off with warm water.

HONEY FACIAL SCRUB RECIPES

18. Honey almond facial scrub

Ingredients:
2 teaspoon ground almonds: for exfoliation
2 teaspoon honey: to moisturize

Direction: Mix the ingredients to form a paste, in a circular motion scrub your face with it and rinse off with warm water. You may increase the quantity for your entire body scrub.

19. Groundnut / Lemon / Honey Facial Scrub

This facial scrub recipe is perfect when you want to moisturize your face, smooth away blemishes and exfoliate your skin gently and naturally.
Ingredients:
Groundnut, Honey and Lemon:

Direction: Stir a couple pinches of ground nuts into a spoonful of honey and a squeeze of lemon juice. The groundnuts are natural exfoliation agents; the lemon juice naturally brightens away blemishes and promotes faster skin growth through its natural acids; and the honey leaves your face smooth, toned and moisturized.

20. Honey Lemon mask for hair removal

Mix together 1teaspoon of lemon juice with 1teaspoon of Honey. Smooth on to the face in the direction of the hair growth and leave on for ten minutes.
Lemon is a natural bleaching and honey a natural soothing agent, therefore the

combination on naturally bleaching hairs works without sensitizing the skin.

21. Honey home made Face lift

Ingredients:
2 heaped teaspoon gram flour (chick pea flour)
½ teaspoon honey
2 teaspoon of water.

Apply it all over the face and neck and leave it on for 15 minutes, use a dampened cotton wool ball or face cloth to wash it off and then moisturize. Because it has a deep cleansing and exfoliating effect, this combination will tighten and soften the skin, making it look vibrant and healthy.

22. Honey mask for spots

2teaspoon honey,
1/4 teaspoon of fine sea salt,
1teaspoon of turmeric.

Blend to a thick paste. Apply only to the spot and leave overnight. Wash your face as normal. This heals the spot faster without leaving scar tissue.

23. Honey spot treatment:

If you're suffering from a breakout, instead of an overly drying over-the-counter pimple cream, why not reach out for ever trusted honey. Apply lightly on the breakout and go to bed, you will awaken to less-stressed skin. If you want a little extra boost, mix the honey with tea tree oil and lavender oil for additional natural cleansing.

Honey facial mask for ACNE:

For skin already suffering from discoloration as a result of breakout scars, honey face masks can help you fade the acne scars and even out skin discoloration, giving you a bright and toned skin. This acne-fighting honey face mask also provides nourishing, exfoliating and cleansing benefits to skin

Ingredients and their importance:

- **Honey**: you already know the importance. Raw honey contains antibacterial properties that remove germs that cause acne from deep within the skin pores.
- **Cinnamon**: Contains potent anti-inflammatory and skin lightening properties.
- **Nutmeg**: has Anti-inflammatory property which helps to reduce swellings and redness from acne and
- **Lemon**: Lemon juice is loaded with vitamin C which is great for skin lightening and removal of acne scars and dark spots
- **Orange:** Rich in vitamin C, orange peel is great for lightening dark spots and acne scars, also evens out skin discolorations.
- **Oats:** Oats not only nourishes skin of all types but also gently exfoliates skin, removing dead cells from the skin surface,

promoting smooth supple skin as well as absorbs excess sebum from within your pores as it is an absorbent.

24.   ACNE Recipe 1

Ingredients:

½ teaspoon cinnamon
1 teaspoon nutmeg
1 teaspoon honey
½ teaspoon lemon juice

Directions:

Mix well all the above ingredients in a small mixing bowl. Using clean finger tips, apply a thick coat of the mixture onto your face. Sit for 15 to 30 minutes to let the face mask settle and get absorbed deep into your skin. Rinse off with warm water and pat dry with a clean towel.

Warning!
Beware of the amount of lemon juice you add to your face mask, more than 8 drops or 1/2 teaspoon will cause a burning sensation

25.   ACNE Recipe 2

Ingredients:

1 teaspoon honey
1 teaspoon orange peel powder
1 teaspoons oats

Directions:

Mix the above ingredients thoroughly in a small mixing bowl apply on your face using clean fingers. Leave on for 15 minutes, rinse your face and pat dry with a clean towel.

26.   *Honey Bee Pollen Face Mask*

This face mask that contains just two ingredients will blow your mind. This is a perfect mask for reduction of wrinkles, skin rejuvenation, toning, nourishing, healing and repairing damaged skin caused by eczema, acne, rashes etc.

Ingredients:
Honey Bee: Packed with vitamins, minerals, amino acids and antioxidants.
Pollen:

Direction:
Rinse the mask away after leaving it on for about 30 minutes to an hour. Apply a few times a week. It's incredibly easy.

CHAPTER THREE

HONEY FOR SKIN CARE:

Honey does wonders to the skin, little wonder why it is found in so many skin-care products in the market today. It acts as an anti-aging agent, as well as moisturizer. It also contains anti-microbial properties and natural antioxidants which help in protecting the skin from sun rays and facilitates the skin's ability to rejuvenate. Apart from that it also refreshes exhausted looking skin, absorb and retain moisture thus leaving it well hydrated, fresh, supple soft and silky. Ancient women were known to use honey and milk to keep their skin youthful, radiant, and smooth.

27.   Smooth Skin Honey Body Lotion

Ingredient:
A spoonful of honey
A teaspoon of organic olive oil
A squeeze of lemon juice

Direction: Stir all the mixtures together, spread on after a bath or whenever your skin needs a little pampering and rinse off with a warm washcloth after 20 minutes.

This skin lotion will moisturize and hydrate your skin, leaving you feeling smooth and soft and the lemon juice which is a natural skin brightener will help fade signs of aging.

28.   Honey Bath Potion
This is the simplest recipe that leaves your skin feeling naturally smooth and soft. Just pour a cup of organic honey into your bath water for a smoothing, hydrating bath experience.

29.   **Honey Body Scrub**.

- You can exfoliate your skin once or twice a week with a gentle scrub made with honey and Baking Soda to remove dead skin cells from their roots and terminating blackheads. Baking soda is known to offer light exfoliation while the honey soothes and smooth the skin, this recipe can be used from head to toe — your arms, legs and feet will also benefit immensely from it. Exfoliation is good for oily as well as dry skin

- Stir a couple pinches of ground nuts into a tablespoon of honey (you can add a squirt of lemon juice). While the ground nuts exfoliate and the lemon juice brightens, the honey will moisturize for a smooth surface

30.   Honey / Lemon & Sugar Scrub

A combination of honey, lemon juice and sugar as body scrub on your skin can work wonders. Mix all three items and scrub gently so you don't bruise your skin, leave it for about 10-15 minutes and rinse with warm water.   Honey cleanses your skin, Lemon juice brightens your skin and sugar is excellent for skin exfoliation.

31.   DRY SKIN BATH

Dry skin can be a lot to deal with during dry winter, but hey, turn to honey to soothe. As the seasons change, in trying to rebalance itself to the conditions, your skin can crack out, but a warm baths with soothing ingredients can keep your skin in check.

Just add two cups of honey to a running bath to create smoothing bliss; soak yourself for 15 minutes, add a cup of Arm & Hammer Baking Soda and soak for another 15 minutes, this will help rid your body of dead skin cells without irritation.

32.   BATH SOAK FOR OTHER SKIN TYPE

Combine 2 tablespoons of honey and 1 cup hot water and let solution dissolve for about 10 minutes. Add 2-3 drops of lavender essential oil, and then pour in bath water. Soak yourself in for at least 20 minutes for a soothing bath.

33.   Honey skin Tanning:

Honey also comes in handy when you want to get rid of tanning due to sun exposure. Mix equal quantities of honey, milk powder, lemon juice and almond oil and apply it on your face, hands, etc. Keep it for 20 minutes and then wash it off.

34. ***Honey Mask for dull look***:
After long hours of outdoor activities the eyes and face will look dull, honey come in handy here

Ingredients:
1 tea spoon honey
½ tea spoon milk
A pinch of saffron powder

Direction: Mix well and apply to face. Wash after 10 min. You could see the glow on your face.

35. HONEY LIP BALM

Ingredient:
1 teaspoon of honey,
½ cup of natural beeswax (grated),
10 drops of lemon essential oil,
2 drops of vitamin E oil
¼ cup of coconut oil.

Direction:

Blend together to obtain an even and creamy paste, scoop into smaller container and you have your lip balm on the go.

36. ***Honey Beeswax Hand cream***:

To make an excellent hand cream against harsh weather condition, mix together a teaspoon of beeswax granules purchased from health food store, with a tablespoon of clear honey, half a teaspoon of olive oil and a few drops of rose essential oil for a soothing, fragrant hand cream.

CHAPTER FOUR

HONEY AND HAIR CARE

Honey is natural and has antibacterial qualities that are beneficial for our skin as well as health. But is honey safe to use on hair? Of course it is! Honey helps retain moisture and gets rid of dry, itchy flakes on the scalp while keeping the hair clean, lustrous, healthy and shiny. The following are some of the honey recipe for hair:

37.   Honey Hair Glow

By infusing honey with your hair cream, it can help make your hair healthy and boost your hair glow. After shampooing, rinse your hair with a mixture of a spoonful of honey with a quart of warm water and leave on for an hour for deep conditioning, then rinse gently. You can also include a rinse of organic apple cider vinegar for extra shine boosting every other week.

For quick rinse, after shampooing your hair, you can add two teaspoons of honey to three cups of water, add some lemon juice, make a mixture of it, rinse your hair with it and dry it normally.

38.   Intensive hair conditioner:

Ingredient:
100g/4oz clear honey
50g/2oz olive oil.

Direction: Mix together thoroughly and massage into damp hair. Wrap your head in a warm towel and relax for 10-15 minutes. Wash hair as normal.

39.   *Hair mask*:

Ingredients:
2 tablespoon Honey,
3 tablespoon olive oil and
1 tablespoon lemon or yoghurt

Heat together the above ingredients and mix well. Warm your hair and apply the mixture to both the scalp and hair. Keep for 30 minutes and then rinse thoroughly.

40.   Hair boost / repair

Adding a teaspoon of honey to your shampoo and using it regularly will give your hair a great boost. Use it normally and let it sit for at least two minutes and then rinse it off. For repair, combine with a teaspoon of olive oil for deeper conditioning. Apply to hair and let soak for 15 minutes and rinse as normal.

41.   **For silky hair and shiny locks**:
If you desire a silky hair, make honey your beauty companion.
Ingredients:
2 tablespoons of curd,
2 eggs,
3 tablespoons of lemon juice
2-3 tablespoons of honey

Direction:
For silky hair mix all ingredients in a bowl and apply it on your scalp and hair, let it sit for 30

minutes and wash off with water. For shiny locks, mix honey with olive oil and apply it on your locks. Let it sit for at least 20 minutes and then wash it off.

Facial hair removal: Facial hair can be a problem but with honey, no problem is without a solution. If getting rid of facial hair is your desire, the following honey home remedy recipes will be beneficial:

42.   Recipe 1
Ingredients:
1 teaspoon of honey
1 tablespoon of sugar
1 teaspoon of lemon juice.

Direction:
In a bowl, mix the ingredients and beat it into a smooth paste, heat it in a microwave for 3 minutes. Make sure it is not too hot; apply it on the area you want to remove the hair in the direction of the hair growth. Take a strip of cloth and place it on top of it and pull it in the opposite direction to remove the hair from the root.

43.   Recipe 2
Ingredients:
1 tablespoon honey
½ tablespoon ground oatmeal
½ teaspoon fresh lemon juice

Direction:
Mix all ingredients into a paste and apply on the face like a mask, let it sit for about 15 minutes

and wash off. For best result do this every other day for up to a month.

44.   *SKIN HAIR WAX*

2 teaspoons of brown sugar,
1 teaspoon of honey
1 teaspoon of water

Mix the above ingredient in a container, heat in the microwave until the mixture turns brown. If it is too thick, add a little water. Let it cool and with a small spatula, apply the wax thinly to skin, with a muslin cloth strip, press and smooth in the direction of hair and then peel back in a swift motion.

45.   *Cinnamon/Honey for scalp condition:*

Having scalp condition in layman's terms means that you have an overgrowth of yeast in your hair which causes your scalp to itch really bad and your hair to fall out in the infected areas. Well all you need is cinnamon and honey paste.

Ingredients:
2 tablespoon of Cinnamon
3 tablespoon Honey
2 teaspoon Cayenne pepper,
2 tablespoon Olive oil,
2 teaspoon Sea salt
3 tablespoon Water.

Direction:
Mix all ingredients and apply to the affected scalp and leave for up to 6 hours and rinse it

then apply only Honey and cinnamon mixture and leave it overnight.

Note: using it for the first time will cause your scalp to tingle and burn a little, after about four hours the burning will stopped.

CHAPTER 5

HONEY Health Drink

46. Honey and Apple Cider Vinegar Health drink:

For cleansing, disinfecting and detoxification of the body the mixture of Honey and Cider Vinegar is second to none. Excellent cleansing agent and natural healing elixir this mixture also contains antibiotic and antiseptic that fights germs and bacteria. It is great for all kinds of allergies and aging. Apple cider vinegar is actually made from fresh, organic, crushed apples that are allowed to mature naturally in wooden barrels, but you can get it easily from the grocery shops or supermarkets

Drinking this mixture can aid in the treatment of the following ailment:

➢ Premature aging
➢ Obesity
➢ Food poisoning
➢ Heat exhaustion
➢ Heartburn
➢ Brittle nails
➢ Bad breath
➢ Arthritis
➢ High blood pressure
➢ High cholesterol level
➢ Eczema

Ingredients
½ to 1 tablespoon of Honey
½ to 1 tablespoon of Apple Cider Vinegar

Direction:
Mix all ingredients in a glass of water and take it once or twice daily.

47.   *Honey and Lemon Drink:*

Drinking lemon juice with a little honey first thing in the morning is an effective anti cellulite treatment as it helps to increase body metabolism.

48.   *Honey and cinnamon drink*

Ingredients:
1 teaspoon Honey,
½ teaspoon Cinnamon powder or ground cinnamon
1 cup boiling Water.

Direction:
Dissolve the cinnamon powder (or ground cinnamon) in a cup of boiling water, stir the mixture and cover for 30 minutes, filter away any big particles and add a teaspoon of honey. Take it first thing in the morning and preferably 30 minutes before breakfast.

49.   *Honey Health shake and energy booster*

Ingredients:

Emergen-C raspberry
Multi-vitamin pack
1 cup water,
¼ finger of banana,
3 fresh strawberries,

3 tablespoons Greek yogurt,
2 tablespoons honey.

Direction: Mix well in blender or handheld high speed mixer. I haven't had a cold in two years, incredible energy boost and actually have lost about ten pounds that I attribute to this shake curbing my appetite an avoiding mid-day snacks.

50.   HONEY AND CINNAMON FOR BAD BREATH

Ingredients:
1 Teaspoon Honey
1/8 Teaspoon Cinnamon Powder
½ cup warm water

Direction: Mix all ingredients and use as a gargle in the morning and in the evening.

51.   Warm Milk & Honey to Treat Conjunctivitis (Pink Eye)

Honey has amazing anti-bacterial properties. Making eyewash with warm milk and honey can help to soothe and treat conjunctivitis. Use equal parts of both honey and milk, making sure the milk is warm (not boiling). Mix together the remedy and keep stirring until the honey becomes smooth in the milk. Use an eyedropper and drop 2-3 drops into your eye several times a day. Alternatively, you can use this mixture as a compress. The anti- bacterial properties in the honey and the soothing effects of the milk will start to work immediately and within 24 hours your pink eye should be cleared up.

www.ingramcontent.com/pod-product-compliance
Lightning Source LLC
Chambersburg PA
CBHW050907290526
45792CB00002B/728